KIDNEY DISEASE COOKBOOK (PESCATARIAN)

Your Best Cook guide to a healthy kidney

Betty May

INTRODUCTION

Welcome to our kidney disease cookbook for pescatarians! In this book, you will find a collection of delicious and nutritious recipes that are tailored to meet the specific dietary needs of individuals with kidney disease who choose to follow a pescatarian lifestyle. Each recipe has been carefully crafted to be low in potassium, phosphorus, and sodium, while still providing essential vitamins and minerals to support overall health. Whether you are new to pescatarian or have been following it for some time, this cookbook offers a wide variety of meal options that are sure to please your taste buds and support your kidney health. So, let's get cooking!"

COPYRIGHT

TABLE OF CONTENT

CHAPTER ONE

Understanding your kidneys and their functions

The kidneys are a set of two organs located in the lower back, on either side of the spine. They play a vital role in maintaining overall health by filtering waste products and excess fluids from the blood, regulating electrolyte balance and blood pressure, and producing hormones that manage red blood cell production and aid bone health.

The kidneys filter the blood through small units called nephrons, which remove waste products and excess fluids in the form of urine. The urine then flows through the ureters, the bladder, and finally out of the body through the urethra.

The kidneys also play a crucial role in regulating electrolyte balance, which is essential for proper nerve and muscle function. They do this by controlling the levels of sodium, potassium, and other electrolytes in the blood.

The kidneys also help moderate blood pressure by releasing a hormone called renin. Renin regulates the production of another hormone called angiotensin, which in turn causes the blood vessels to constrict, thereby increasing blood pressure.

The kidneys also produce a hormone called erythropoietin, which regulates the production of red blood cells in the bone marrow. This hormone is essential for maintaining adequate oxygen levels in the body.

In addition, the kidneys produce a hormone called calcitriol, which helps the body absorb calcium and promote healthy bone growth.

What is a Chronic Kidney Disease?

Chronic kidney disease is a continuous loss of kidney function over time. It can be caused by different factors, including high blood pressure, diabetes, and infections. Symptoms of CKD include fatigue, swelling, and difficulty sleeping. If left untreated, CKD can lead to end-stage renal disease (ESRD), which requires dialysis or a kidney transplant to survive.

It is important to maintain a healthy lifestyle to prevent kidney disease and other kidney-related problems. This includes eating a healthy diet, maintaining a healthy weight, exercising regularly, and controlling blood pressure and blood sugar levels. It is also important to get regular checkups and screenings to detect any potential kidney problems early on.

CHAPTER TWO

Causes and Symptoms

kidney disease develops over time if kidney harm progresses sluggishly. Loss of kidney function can result in a buildup of fluid or body waste or electrolyte problems. Depending on how severe it is, loss of order function can cause

- Nausea
- Vomiting
- Loss of appetite
- Fatigue and weakness
- Sleep problems
- Urinating more or less
- reduced cerebral sharpness
- Muscle cramps
- Swelling of feet and ankles
- Dry, itchy skin
- High blood pressure(hypertension) that is delicate to control

- the abruptness of breath, if fluid builds up in the lungs
- Chest pain

These signs are frequently nonspecific. meaning they can also be caused by other ails. Because your kidneys are capable of making up for lost function, you might not develop signs and symptoms until unrecoverable damage has happened.

causes of kidney disease include

- Type 1 or type 2 diabetes
- High blood pressure
- Swelling of the kidney's filtering units
- Interstitial nephritis is an inflammation of the kidney's tubules and enclosing structures
- Polycystic kidney disease or other inherited kidney conditions
- extended interference of the urinary tract, from conditions similar to an enlarged prostate, kidney stones, and some cancers

CHAPTER THREE

Diet and nutrition for kidney disease.

Diet and nutrition play a critical role in managing and preventing kidney disease. Eating a healthy diet can help slow down the progression of the disease, control symptoms, and improve overall health.

In kidney disease, the kidneys are not able to filter waste products and excess fluids as efficiently as they should. This can result in a buildup of toxins in the body, which can be harmful. A healthy diet can help reduce the load on the kidneys and prevent further damage.

Here are some dietary recommendations for individuals with kidney disease:

- Limit protein intake: Excess protein can put a strain on the kidneys and increase the risk of further damage. It is recommended to limit protein intake to the recommended daily allowance (RDA) for protein, which is about 0.8 grams of protein per kilogram of body weight per day.
- Control sodium and potassium intake: Sodium and potassium are electrolytes that need to be in balance for the body to function properly. Individuals with kidney disease may need to limit their intake of these nutrients, as the kidneys may not be able to effectively regulate their levels in the body.
- Limit phosphorus: High levels of phosphorus in the blood can lead to a condition called hyperphosphatemia, which can cause bones to become weak and brittle. It is recommended to

limit the intake of foods high in phosphorus, such as dairy products, meat, and processed foods.

- Drink plenty of water: Staying hydrated is important for overall health and can help prevent dehydration, which can be harmful to individuals with kidney disease.
- Limit fluids: In advanced stages of kidney disease, the body may retain fluids, leading to swelling and discomfort. In these cases, it may be necessary to limit fluid intake to prevent further fluid buildup.
- Eat a balanced diet: A balanced diet that includes plenty of fruits, vegetables, whole grains, and lean proteins can provide the nutrients needed for overall health and help manage the symptoms of kidney disease.

It is important to follow a healthcare provider and a dietitian to create a personalised diet and nutrition plan, as each individual's needs may be different based on their stage of kidney disease, medications, and other health conditions.

A healthy diet and nutrition are critical components in managing and preventing kidney disease.

What to Eat and What to Avoid

A pescatarian diet that is specifically designed for individuals with kidney disease can be beneficial in slowing down the progression of the disease and controlling symptoms. To effectively manage kidney disease through diet, it is important to understand what foods to include and what to avoid.

Here is a list of foods to eat and avoid in a kidney disease pescatarian cookbook:

Foods to eat:

- Fish and seafood: Fish and seafood are good sources of lean protein, which is essential for overall health. Choose low-mercury fish, such as salmon, tilapia, and cod, and avoid high-mercury fish, such as swordfish, shark, and tilefish.
- Fruits and vegetables: Fruits and vegetables are low in sodium and high in fibre, vitamins, and minerals. It is important to include a variety of colourful fruits and vegetables in your diet to ensure a wide range of nutrients.
- Whole grains: Whole grains are an excellent source of fibre and provide a variety of essential vitamins and minerals. Choose whole-grain bread, pasta, rice, and other grains instead of refined grains.
- Legumes: Legumes, such as beans, lentils, and chickpeas, are a good source of plant-based protein, fibre,

and a variety of essential vitamins and minerals.

Foods to avoid:

- High-protein foods: Foods high in protein, such as meat, poultry, dairy products, and eggs, can put a strain on the kidneys and increase the risk of further damage.
- Sodium-rich foods: Sodium can cause fluid retention and raise blood pressure, which can be harmful to individuals with kidney disease. Foods to avoid include processed foods, canned soups, and snacks.
- High-potassium foods: High potassium levels can be harmful to individuals with kidney disease, as the kidneys may not be able to effectively regulate potassium levels in the body. Foods to avoid include bananas, oranges, potatoes, and tomato sauce.

- High-phosphorus foods: High levels of phosphorus in the blood can lead to a condition called hyperphosphatemia, which can cause bones to become weak and brittle. Foods to avoid include dairy products, meat, and processed foods.

CHAPTER FOUR

Purpose of this cookbook.

A pescatarian cookbook is a collection of recipes that cater to individuals who follow a pescatarian diet. This type of diet includes fish and seafood as a source of protein but excludes meat, poultry, and other animal products such as dairy and eggs.

The purpose of a pescatarian cookbook is to provide individuals with a variety of delicious and nutritious meal options that align with their dietary restrictions. It offers a range of recipes that incorporate a variety of ingredients and cooking styles, allowing for a well-rounded and satisfying pescatarian diet.

There are several benefits to following a pescatarian diet and using a pescatarian cookbook:

- Increased consumption of healthy fats: Fish and seafood are rich in healthy fats, such as omega-3 fatty acids, which have been shown to have a variety of health benefits, including reducing the risk of heart disease, depression, and inflammation.
- Better heart health: A pescatarian diet that includes a variety of fish and seafood has been linked to a lower risk of heart disease and stroke, due to the high levels of heart-healthy fats and low levels of saturated fats.
- Improved mental health: The omega-3 fatty acids found in fish have been shown to have a positive impact on mental health, including reducing the risk of depression and improving cognitive function.

- Increased nutrient intake: A pescatarian diet that includes a variety of fruits, vegetables, whole grains, and legumes provides a wealth of essential vitamins and minerals, including vitamins C and D, folate, and iron.
- Environmental sustainability: A pescatarian diet that includes fish and seafood can be more environmentally sustainable than a diet that includes meat, poultry, and other animal products. This is because fish and seafood have a lower carbon footprint and require less land and water to produce compared to other animal products.

This pescatarian cookbook provides individuals with a collection of delicious and nutritious meal options that align with their dietary restrictions. The benefits of a pescatarian diet include increased consumption of healthy fats, better heart health, improved mental health, increased nutrient intake, and environmental sustainability. Whether an individual has chosen a pescatarian diet for health, ethical, or environmental reasons, this pescatarian cookbook can help them make delicious and well-rounded meals.

CHAPTER FIVE

Recipes

These pescatarian recipes are simple to prepare and provide a delicious and nutritious meal option for individuals who follow a pescatarian diet. They incorporate a variety of ingredients and cooking styles, making it easy to enjoy a well-rounded and satisfying meal.

Here are some simple and delicious pescatarian recipes that can be prepared at home:

Grilled Salmon with Lemon and Herbs:

Ingredients:

4 salmon fillets

4 tablespoons olive oil

2 lemons, juiced

4 garlic cloves, minced
2 tablespoons chopped fresh herbs (such as basil, thyme, and parsley)
Salt and pepper, to taste

Instructions:
Preheat the grill to medium-high heat.
In a small bowl, mix the olive oil, lemon juice, minced garlic, herbs, salt, and pepper.
Place the salmon fillets on a large piece of aluminium foil and brush the lemon and herb mixture onto both sides of the fish.
Wrap the foil around the salmon fillets, making a sealed packet.
Place the foil packet on the grill and cook for 10-12 minutes, or until the fish is cooked through.
Serve the grilled salmon with lemon wedges and a side of roasted vegetables or whole-grain rice.

Baked Tilapia with Pesto and Tomatoes:

Ingredients:

4 tilapia fillets
4 tablespoons basil pesto
4 ripe tomatoes, sliced
Salt and pepper, to taste
Fresh basil leaves, for garnish

Instructions:
Preheat the oven to 400°F (200°C).
Make a big baking sheet with parchment paper.
Put the tilapia fillets on the baking sheet.
Spread 2 tablespoons of pesto onto each fillet.
Top each fillet with sliced tomatoes and sprinkle with salt and pepper.
Bake for 15-20 minutes, or until the fish is cooked through and the tomatoes are slightly roasted.
Serve the baked tilapia with a side of roasted vegetables or whole-grain pasta.

Cod and Vegetable Stir-Fry:
Ingredients:

1 pound cod fillet, cut into bite-sized pieces
1 tablespoon olive oil
1 red bell pepper, sliced
1 yellow onion, sliced
2 garlic cloves, minced
1 cup sliced mushrooms
1 cup snow peas
2 tablespoons low-sodium soy sauce
2 tablespoons rice vinegar
1 teaspoon cornstarch
Fresh cilantro leaves, for garnish

Instructions:
Heat the olive oil in a large skillet over high heat.
Add the sliced red bell pepper, yellow onion, minced garlic, sliced mushrooms, and snow peas. Stir-fry for 2-3 minutes, or until the vegetables are slightly softened.
Add the cod pieces to the wok and continue to stir-fry for another 2-3 minutes, or until the fish is cooked through.
In a small bowl, whisk together the soy sauce, rice vinegar, and cornstarch.

Pour the sauce mixture over the stir-fry and continue to stir until the sauce thickens. Serve the cod and vegetable stir-fry over a bed of brown rice and garnish with fresh cilantro leaves.

Pesto Pasta with Shrimp -

Ingredients

10 ounces of dry spaghetti can also use linguine or fettuccine

3/4 cup basil pesto

1 pound medium to large shrimp peeled and deveined

1 tablespoon olive oil

1 teaspoon Italian seasoning (or equal parts garlic powder dried basil and dried oregano)

salt and pepper to taste

1/4 cup parmesan cheese

1 cup cherry tomatoes halved

Optional garnish: chopped parsley

Instructions

Put a large pot of salted water to a boil, and cook the pasta according to package directions.
While the pasta is cooking, prepare the shrimp.
In a pan, Heat the olive oil over high heat. Add the shrimp and sprinkle with Italian seasoning, salt, and pepper.
Cook for 2-4 minutes or until shrimp is just pink and opaque. Turn off the heat.
Drain the pasta and add it to the pan with the shrimp. Stir in the pesto.
Add the cherry tomatoes and parmesan cheese to the pan. Garnish with chopped parsley if desired.

Fish Tacos

Ingredients

- 3 tbsp. extra-virgin olive oil
- Juice of 1 lime
- 2 tsp. chilli powder
- 1 tsp. paprika
- 1/2 tsp. ground cumin

- 1/2 tsp. cayenne pepper
- 1 1/2 lb. cod (or other flaky white fish)
- 1/2 tbsp. vegetable oil
- salt
- Freshly ground black pepper
- 8 corn tortillas
- 1 avocado, diced
- Lime wedges, for serving
- Sour cream, for serving

Ingredients

- Bake or grill your choice of fish fillets, then serve with shredded lettuce, diced tomatoes, and avocado mixed in the sour cream in a corn tortilla.

Seafood Paella -

Ingredients

- 4 1/2 cups chicken stock
- 1/2 teaspoon saffron threads, crumbled and then loosely measured
- 1/4 teaspoon salt
- 3 tablespoons olive oil
- 1/2 yellow onion, finely chopped
- 1/2 red bell pepper, finely chopped
- 3 cloves garlic, finely chopped
- 6 ounces mild dried chorizo sausage, sliced into thin half-moons
- 3 cups short-grain rice, such as Spanish Bomba rice or Italian Arborio
- 1 (14-ounce) can of fire-roasted diced tomatoes
- 1 cup frozen green peas

- 1 pound large (21-24 per pound) shrimp, peeled and deveined, with tails left on

- 1-pound mussels, rinsed and scrubbed

- 1 pound littleneck clams, rinsed and scrubbed

- 1/4 cup chopped parsley, for garnish

Instructions

Heat a gas grill to medium-high heat (375°F), in a saucepan over medium heat, and bring the stock to a boil. Add the saffron and salt. Put off the heat and allow the saffron to steep for at least 15 minutes. Taste and add more salt, if needed. In pan **Sauté** onions, garlic, and diced red pepper, then add arborio rice, diced tomatoes, saffron, and white wine. Add in clams, mussels, and shrimp, then bake in the oven until the seafood is cooked through and the rice is tender.

Tuna Stuffed Avocado

Ingredients

4 avocados

2 5-ounce cans of tuna (I prefer albacore tuna)

1/4 cup mayonnaise

1 stalk of celery, diced
2 tbsp red onion, diced
1-2 tbsp chopped parsley, chives, and/or other herbs

1/2 tbsp mustard

salt and pepper, to taste

Instructions

Mix canned tuna with mayonnaise, lemon juice, and diced onion, then stuff the mixture into a ripe avocado half.

Shrimp Scampi -

Ingredients

4 garlic cloves, 2 grated, 2 thinly sliced

1 teaspoon salt

3 tablespoons olive oil, divided

1 pound large shrimp, peeled, deveined

¼ teaspoon red pepper flakes

¼ cup dry white wine

1 tablespoon fresh lemon juice

½ stick unsalted butter

3 tablespoons chopped parsley

Warm crusty bread for serving

Instructions

Whisk grated garlic, salt, and 1 Tbsp. oil in a medium bowl. Add shrimp and stir for at least 10 minutes

Heat remaining 2 Tbsp. oil in a large pan over medium heat and cook shrimp mixture until shrimp is pink but still slightly underdone, leaving as much oil in the pan as possible. Add sliced garlic and red pepper to the pan and cook, tossing, until fragrant, about 1 minute. Add wine and lemon juice and cook, stirring occasionally, for about 2 minutes. Add butter and cook until butter is melted and sauce is thickened, about 5 minutes more. Scrape shrimp along with any accumulated juices into a skillet. Toss to coat and cook until shrimp are fully cooked. Transfer to a plate, top with parsley, and serve with bread for dipping.

Fish and Chips -

Ingredients

- 500 gm fish fillets
- 250 gm potato
- 1 egg
- salt as required
- 1/2 cup breadcrumbs
- 1 cup all-purpose flour
- 1 teaspoon baking powder
- 1 cup milk
- black pepper as required
- 2 cups refined oil

Instructions

Cut potato in fries and prepare the batter for frying fish. wash and peel the potatoes. Cut them into fries, and keep them aside in salted water. Take a deep-bottomed mixing bowl and mix together all-purpose flour, milk, egg, baking powder, salt & pepper. Prepare a thick batter and keep it aside for 15 minutes. gently add the fish fillets to the prepared batter and coat them well with it.

Then coat them well in the breadcrumbs. Take a frying pan, keep it on medium flame, and add refined oil to it. Deep fry the coated fish until golden brown from both sides. Take a pan and keep it on medium flame and heat oil in it. Deep fry the fries in the pan. Once done, serve with the fried fish fillets and enjoy!

Shrimp and Grits

Ingredients

- 4 1/2 cups water

- 1 teaspoon salt

- 1 cup stone-ground white grits

- 2 tablespoons unsalted butter

- 2 ounces white cheddar cheese, shredded

- 4 thick slices of bacon

- 1 cup chopped white or yellow onion

- 1 cup chopped green pepper

- 2 cloves garlic, minced

- 1 to 1 1/2 pounds of shrimp, peeled and deveined

- 1 cup chicken stock

- 3 green onions

- 2 tablespoons chopped parsley

- 2 tbsp lemon juice.

Instruction

Fry the bacon in a pan on medium heat until crispy. Remove and chop. Boil some water in a medium pot. Add the salt. pour the grits into the boiling water while you stir with a wooden spoon so you don't get any lumps. When all the grits are incorporated, lower the heat and cook the grits for 35 minutes stirring frequently. Reserve about some of the shrimp whole and cut the rest into 3 to 4 pieces each. Set aside.When the grits have cooked for 30 minutes, heat the pan on medium-high. sauté the onion and green pepper over medium-high heat until soft, about 4 minutes.Add the bacon, garlic cloves and shrimp and toss to combine. Let this cook another minute.Add the chicken stock and let this boil down for 5 minutes.Then stir the cheddar cheese and butter into the grits. Serve together at once.

Baked Tilapia with Tomato and Olive Topping -

Ingredients

- 4 (6-ounce) tilapia fillets

- ¼ teaspoon salt
- ¼ teaspoon freshly ground black pepper
- Cooking spray
- 1 cup cherry tomatoes, halved
- ¾ cup pitted green olives, coarsely chopped
- 3 tablespoons chopped fresh flat-leaf parsley
- 3 garlic cloves, minced

Instructions

Preheat the oven to 375°.Sprinkle salt and pepper in the fish. coate pan with cooking spray and arrange the fish. Combine tomatoes and remaining ingredients; toss gently. Arrange tomato mixture around fish on baking sheet.Bake at 375° for 20 minutes until fish flakes easily when tested with a fork or as preferred. Serve topping each serving with about 1/4 cup tomato mixture.

Ceviche -

Ingredients

1. Shrimp
2. 3 Limes
3. 2 Lemons
4. Roma tomatoes
5. Red onions
6. Cilantro
7. Jalapeno: If you like it less spicy remove the seeds
8. Salt and pepper
9. Cucumber

10.   Avocado

Instructions

Boil water in pot, fill another bowl with ice water: Add shrimp to boiling water and let cook just until pink for about a minute.Drain, chill it in the bowl of ice water for 10 minutes then chop shrimp. In a bowl combine shrimp, lime juice, lemon juice, tomatoes, onion, cilantro, jalapeno pepper and season with salt and pepper to taste.Marinate: Transfer to refrigerator and let rest for 1 hour.Toss in cucumber and avocado and serve with tortilla chips

Sardines on Toast -
Ingredients

- 2 slices white or brown bread
- 1 tin sardines (in brine or oil)
- Butter
- Black Pepper
- Lemon juice(lemon juice)

Instructions

- Toast the bread in the toaster.
- Butter the toast.
- Open the sardine tin and drain the oil or water from the can.
- Add sardines to the toast and mash a bit on the top.
- Garnish to preference with black pepper and/or a squirt of lemon juice.

Calamari Salad

Ingredients

1 1/2 lb cleaned squid

2 tablespoons fresh lemon juice

1 tablespoon red-wine vinegar

1/3 cup extra-virgin olive oil

1 large garlic clove, minced

1/2 teaspoon salt

1/4 teaspoon black pepper

1 small red onion, halved lengthwise, then thinly sliced crosswise (1 cup)

1/3 cup pitted Kalamata olives, halved lengthwise

2 cups cherry or grape tomatoes (3/4 lb), halved or quartered if large

2 celery ribs, cut into 1/4-inch-thick slices

1 cup loosely packed fresh flat-leaf parsley leaves.

Instructions

Rinse squid under cold running water, then lightly pat dry with paper towels. Halve tentacles lengthwise and cut bodies crosswise into 1/3-inch-wide rings.

Cook squid in a 5- to 6-quart pot of salted boiling water, uncovered, until just opaque, 40 to 60 seconds. Drain and immediately transfer to a bowl of ice and cold water to stop cooking. When the squid is cool, drain and pat dry.

Whisk together lemon juice, vinegar, oil, garlic, salt, and pepper in a small bowl, then stir in onion and let stand for 5 minutes.Combine squid, olives, tomatoes, celery, and parsley in a large bowl. Toss with dressing and season with salt and pepper. Let sir at least 15 minutes to allow flavours to develop. Cook calamari rings until tender, then toss with mixed greens, cherry tomatoes, and balsamic vinaigrette.

Spicy Shrimp Linguine -
Ingredients

3 tablespoons olive oil
4 garlic cloves, smashed
1/2 teaspoon red pepper flakes
2 teaspoons sun-dried tomato paste*
1 (14.5-ounce) can no salt added diced tomatoes
2 tablespoons white wine**
16 ounces bite-size shrimp, peeled and deveined, tails removed
1 tablespoon butter
1/4 cup flat-leaf parsley, chopped
4 ounces whole-grain linguine or spaghetti
black pepper to taste.

Instructions

Bring a large stock pot of water to boil, and prepare the pasta according to package directions, omitting salt.

In a skillet, heat olive oil over medium heat. Add the garlic and red pepper flakes. When the garlic starts to sizzle, stir in the sun-dried tomato paste.

Add the diced tomatoes, and cook over low heat for 15 minutes, stirring occasionally.

Add wine and cook for 1 minute.
Cook shrimp until pink.
Remove the pan from heat and stir in the butter.Drain pasta and place in warmed Top with shrimp mixture and parsley.
Serves 4 (1/2 c cooked pasta, 3 oz shrimp and 1/2 c sauce).
 Cook linguine according to package instructions, then toss with sautéed garlic, red pepper flakes, diced tomatoes, and cooked shrimp.

Sole with Lemon Butter Sauce

Ingredients

lemon sole fillet or whole fish
4 tbsp plain flour
1 tsp salt and pepper each
4-5 tbsp unsalted butter
1 lemon
2 tbsp capers
1 tbsp chopped fresh parsley

Instructions

In a large bowl combine the flour, salt and pepper. Dredge the fish in the flour mixture, then shake off the excess flour.
Preheat a frying pan and melt 2 tbsp of butter in it. Fry the sole in butter for approximately 2 minutes on each side. Then remove from the pan and keep warm.
On the same pan add the remaining butter and watch it turn slightly brown, then add the juice of half a lemon and slices of the other half, cook for a few seconds, then add the capers and return the fish back to the pan. Spread the sauce all over the fish and take off the heat. sprinkle with fresh parsley.

Squid Stir-Fry

Ingredients

For the sauce
1 tsp of cornstarch
1 tbsp of Chinese cooking wine
1 tbsp of soy sauce
2 tbsp of oyster sauce
1 tbsp of water
1 tsp of sugar

1 tsp of black pepper
1 tsp of dark soy sauce for the colour
For stir fry
12 ounces of squid
Few slices of ginger for blanching the squid
2 tbsp of oil to stir-fry
Some ginger strips
3 cloves of minced garlic
Some white part of spring onion
1/2 of red bell pepper
1/2 of green bell pepper

Instructions

Clean the squid and remove the skin.
use your knife to create some patterns on
the squid so it will look better and be more
tender. Make sure the inside part is facing
up. Run your knife gently and evenly but
don't cut off. Switch an angle, do the same
thing again. Then cut the squid into small
pieces.
Also, cut the wings the same way and cut the
tentacles into small pieces.

Next, we will quickly blanch the squid. Prepare a pot of water. Add a few slices of ginger. Bring the water to a boil. My rule for cooking squid is – eight it is less than 2 minutes or more than 2 hours. Anytime between that, it is going to be tough. So we will just put this in for only 10 seconds. This is just to remove the bad smell. Then quickly take it out. Rinse the squid under cold water and drain it completely.

Now let's make the sauce (1 tsp of cornstarch, 1 tbsp of Chinese cooking wine, 1 tbsp of soy sauce, 2 tbsp of oyster sauce, 1 tbsp of water, 1 tsp of sugar, 1 tsp of black pepper, 1 tsp of dark soy sauce)

Mix that up and the sauce is done. Let's start cooking.

Turn the heat to high, add 2 tbsp of oil. Wait for the wok to get hot. Add some ginger strips, garlic, white part of spring onion. Stir this until fragrant.

Add the bell pepper. Stir them for about 3 minutes or whenever you think the pepper is ready.

Add in the squid. Remember I said, we need to cook the squid in less than 2 minutes. We already blanch the squid for 10 seconds, now you only have 1 minute and 50 seconds left. Make sure you use the highest heat possible. This is the key to a Chinese stir-fry dish. Everything needs to cook really fast in the wok. If you use low heat, it will take longer to cook and the food will start producing water which you don't want. Add the sauce 20 seconds before you turn off the heat. Toss everything together. Count the time correctly and you can take it out. Serve it with white rice.

Tofu and Veggie Frittata

Ingredients

1 package (350 g) firm tofu, drained
¾ cup aquafaba (from cooked/canned chickpea)
¼ cup + 2 tbsp chickpea flour or all-purpose flour
1 medium potato, diced (1 cup)
1 medium red bell pepper, diced (1 cup)

1 large zucchini, diced (2 cups)
4 green onions, sliced (1 cup)
¼ cup cilantro, finely
2 tbsp nutritional yeast
1.5 tbsp miso
1 tbsp garlic powder
1 tbsp onion powder
¼ tsp turmeric
¼ tsp sea salt
1 tsp red pepper flakes (adjust as needed)

Instructions

Preheat the oven to 350 °F.

In a blender, combine tofu, aquafaba (liquid from canned or cooked chickpea), flour, nutritional yeast, miso, garlic powder, onion powder, turmeric, sea salt, and red pepper flakes into a smooth batter.

Dice red bell pepper, potato, and zucchini into small pieces. Finely chop green onions and cilantro.

Add diced bell pepper and potatoes to a pan and sauté for about 10 minutes, until the potatoes are cooked.

Add zucchini, green onions, and cilantro and mix well. Sauté until vegetables are tender, about 5 minutes.

Transfer the cooked vegetables into an 8-inch pie dish. Pour the batter over the vegetables and mix well.

Bake for 60 minutes until the top of the frittata browns. Remove from the oven and let it cool for a few minutes. Slice and serve.

Hake and Potato Stew

Ingredients

Extra virgin olive oil
6 hake fillets
2 tablespoons flour
1 chopped onion
3 leeks, sliced
2 potatoes, clicked
1 teaspoon tomato paste
A pinch of sweet paprika
Fish soup
2 boiled eggs
Chopped fresh parsley
Sal Island

Black pepper

Instructions

Season the tenderloins of hake and we pass them through flour to then fry them in a saucepan with a good jet of oil. When they have browned, we take them out and reserve them.

In the same pot, sauté the onion for 5 minutes.

Then we add the leek, season and fry the whole for 10 minutes, until the vegetables are very soft.

Then, we incorporate the potatoes into pieces and sauté for a couple of minutes before adding the concentrated tomato, the paprika and the fish stock, which should cover the whole.

We return the hake to the casserole and we cook for approximately 15 minutes until the potatoes are tender.

To finish, decorate with the boiled egg and sliced and chopped parsley and give a few wiggles to the casserole.

Tuna Noodle Caboodle

Ingredients

1 tin of Scout Tuna in Olive Oil
1 pinch of salt
2 cups of elbow macaroni
¼ cups of salted butter
¼ cups of all purpose flour
2 tbs of Old Bay seasoning
2 cups of whole milk
2 cups of mozzarella or provolone cheese
½ cup of frozen corn
½ cup of frozen peas
½ cup of frozen carrots
1 bag of Covered Bridge chips, or a crunchy chip of your choice

Instructions

Preheat your oven to 350 degrees.
Bring a medium sized pot of water to a boil.
Add a pinch of salt and cook the macaroni noodles until they're very, very tender (15-20 minutes).

In another medium sized pot, melt your butter on low-medium heat and whisk in your flour.
When a nice almond colour begins to develop, add in your Old Bay seasoning and whole milk. Whisk everything together and increase the heat to medium-high. The sauce will begin to thicken.
Once your sauce has thickened, melt in all your cheese. Set aside.
Mix together your cheese sauce, noodles, corn, peas, carrots and Scout Tuna in Olive Oil into an oven-proof casserole dish.
Bake for 30 minutes, or until the top is bubbling and golden.
Remove your casserole from the oven, and crumble your chips on top. Serve hot

Haddock and broccoli bake

Ingredients
2 tbsp olive oil
½ tbs smoked paprika
A pinch ground turmeric
2 tbsp wheat (cake) flour

625 ml warm low-fat milk

1 t fish spice

flaked sea salt and fresh black pepper, to taste

60 ml grated parmesan cheese, optional

60 ml grated mozzarella cheese, plus 30 ml extra

60 ml grated mature cheddar cheese, plus 30 ml extra

500 g fresh or frozen MSC certified haddock, cut into chunks

400 g long stem broccoli stems

1 teaspoon freshly ground black pepper

Instructions

Preheat the roaster to 180° C. In a saucepan, heat the olive oil, add the spices and cook for 30 seconds.Whisk in the flour a little at a time to cause a roux. Remove the pan off the heat and whisk in the warm milk. Place the pan back on the heat and continue whisking until the sauce thickens.

Bring to the boil and poach for 8 minutes, still whisking. Season the fish with preferred

spice, salt and pepper and stir until well combined.
Switch off the cookstove and add the different cheeses, stir until melted. Pour the sauce into a roaster- proof baking dish.
Place the fused and stroke- dried haddock chunks on top of the sauce followed by broccoli stems. season the broccoli with a pinch of salt. Sprinkle it with the spare cheddar and mozzarella cheese.
Bake in the roaster for 20 minutes until the fish is cooked and the sauce is golden. Serve with fresh dill and lime wedges and starch of your choice(similar as crusty bread, potatoes, or fries).

I hope you enjoy these pescatarian recipes!

CHAPTER SIX

SUMMARY

In conclusion, a pescatarian kidney disease cookbook is a comprehensive guide that is designed to support individuals with kidney disease in their quest for better health through nutrition. The pescatarian diet, which includes fish and other seafood but eliminates meat and poultry, is a nutritious and delicious way to manage kidney health. The recipes and tips included in this cookbook are carefully crafted to meet the unique dietary needs of individuals with kidney disease, ensuring that they can enjoy a balanced and flavorful diet while taking care of their health.

The pescatarian diet is ideal for individuals with kidney disease because it is naturally low in phosphorus, which is a nutrient that can be harmful to the kidneys in high amounts. Phosphorus is found in many foods, including meat and poultry, but is abundant in fish and other seafood. By including more fish and seafood in the diet and limiting other sources of phosphorus, individuals with kidney disease can help support their kidney function and reduce the risk of further damage.

In addition to being low in phosphorus, the pescatarian diet is also high in protein, a nutrient that is essential for building and repairing tissues in the body. Fish and other seafood are excellent sources of high-quality protein, and can provide the essential amino acids that the body needs to function properly. By including plenty of fish and seafood in their diets, individuals with kidney disease can help support their overall health and well-being.

This cookbook includes a variety of recipes that are not only nutritious and delicious, but also easy to prepare. From flavorful seafood stews and soups to tasty fish tacos and grilled salmon, there is something for everyone. Each recipe is accompanied by detailed nutritional information, so that individuals with kidney disease can make informed decisions about their food choices. In conclusion, a pescatarian kidney disease cookbook is a comprehensive guide to better health through nutrition. By following a pescatarian diet and using the recipes in this cookbook, individuals with kidney disease can feel confident in their food choices, enjoy a balanced and flavorful diet, and support their overall health and well-being.